Unraveling the Emotions of Missing You:

Navigating Longing, Healing Hearts, and Rediscovering Love.

Table of contents

Introduction

In a quiet corner of the city, where the streets were lined with nostalgia and the breeze whispered secrets of forgotten stories, lived Rosa T. Skelton. She was a woman of quiet grace, and her eyes held a world of experiences that only those who dared to listen closely could fathom. Her days were woven with threads of memories, and her heart carried the weight of longing that had taken root years ago.

Rosa had always been a keen observer of emotions, a weaver of words, and a collector of moments. Her home was filled with trinkets that held stories—faded photographs, handwritten letters, and a worn leather journal that chronicled the chapters of her life. But it was the chapter titled "Missing You" that she turned to most often.

The story began many summers ago, a time when laughter echoed through the streets and the sun painted the world in hues of gold. Rosa had met Alex under the shade of an old oak tree, their hearts finding resonance in the cadence of each other's laughter. From that moment on, their lives seemed to intertwine effortlessly, like two melodies harmonizing into one beautiful symphony.

Alex had a spirit as vibrant as the sunrise, and his absence was an ache that lingered like the last note of a song. He was a traveler, a seeker of new horizons, and his wanderlust had carried him across oceans and continents. Each time he left, Rosa's heart held both the promise of his return and the uncertainty of when it would come to fruition

As the years passed, Rosa and Alex's connection evolved into a tapestry of emotions: the joy of shared moments, the sadness of farewells, and the anticipation of reunions. The pages of Rosa's leather journal chronicled it all—the laughter, the tears, the letters exchanged, and the long nights spent under the stars, imagining each other's presence.

The journal was Rosa's sanctuary, a place where she poured out her heart, unraveled her thoughts, and explored the intricate labyrinth of emotions that missing someone entails. It became a testament to the depth of human connection and the resilience of the heart in the face of absence.

One winter's day, as snowflakes danced outside her window, Rosa received a letter from Alex. The words danced across the page, carrying with them the scent of distant lands and the warmth of shared memories. He wrote of new landscapes, of friendships forged, and of dreams realized. And as Rosa read his words, she felt a curious sensation—a bittersweet blend of joy for his adventures and a pang of longing for his presence.

It was then that Rosa realized the power of missing someone and how it could be a catalyst for growth, a source of inspiration, and a reminder of the beauty that exists in the spaces between moments. She understood that missing someone wasn't just a void to be filled; it was a canvas upon which memories painted their colors, emotions textures, and time its intricate patterns.

As Rosa continued to write in her journal, her words began to take on a life of their own. She crafted poems that captured the essence of missing someone: the ache, the yearning, and the whispered hopes for the future. Her journal transformed into a treasure trove of emotions, a testament to the resilience of the heart and the bonds that transcend distance.

In the quiet hours of the night, Rosa would often sit by her window, gazing at the stars and feeling the presence of Alex in every twinkling light. She had come to understand that missing someone was not a sign of weakness; it was a testament to the strength of the love they shared. Even though she was still grieving his loss, she was also thankful for the time they shared, the memories they made, and the love that united them.

And so, in the cozy corner of the city where the streets whispered stories and the wind carried echoes of longing, Rosa T. Skelton continued to unravel the emotions of missing you, a journey that had transformed her heart, enriched her soul, and taught her that even in absence, love had the power to bridge the spaces between two souls.

The Feelings of Missing Someone

1. Yearning: A strong yearning is at the center of missing someone. It's a need to be close to them, to feel their presence, and to bask in the warmth of their companionship once more. This longing can result in a throb that is both sweet and terrible, aiding us in remembering the value of the relationships we cherish.

2. Sentimentality: Missing somebody frequently sets off a surge of emotions. Sentimentality washes over us, conveying with it pictures of shared minutes, giggling, and the excellence of times past. These recollections give solace, yet they can likewise heighten the longing to remember those esteemed encounters.

3. Misery: The shortcomings of somebody we care about can prompt a significant feeling of bitterness. This feeling results from the void they leave behind and the knowledge that we cannot relive those moments exactly as they were.

The misery of their shortcomings is a powerful sign of their effect on our lives.

4. Weakness: Missing someone can leave us feeling sincerely uncovered. The desire for association can make us feel powerless and vulnerable to our emotions. This weakness can be awkward, but it can also be an impetus for self-disclosure and development.

5. Confinement: In this situation, we could feel detached, as though a piece of our day-to-day schedule or emotionally supportive network is absent. This segregation can increase our yearning and help us remember the interconnectedness that improves our lives.

6. Trust: Amid the hurt of missing somebody, there is often a promise of something better. Trust for future reunions, discussions, and shared encounters keeps the soul alive and the heart open.

7. Reflection: Missing someone can provoke profound thoughtfulness. We think about the significance of the relationship, the lessons learned, and the effect they've had on forming our identity.

8. Appreciation: The shortcomings of somebody we care for can enhance our appreciation for their presence. We come to figure out the meaning of their part in our lives and perceive the characteristics that make them special and esteemed.

9. Compassion: Encouraging feelings of missing somebody can cultivate sympathy toward other people who may be going through comparable sentiments. This common experience can reinforce associations with companions, family, and outsider.

Chapter 1.

The Idea of Association

Individuals are intrinsically friendly animals, wired for association, sympathy, and friendship. The idea of our associations with others is an embroidery woven from strings of shared encounters, common comprehension, and close-to-home reverberation. These associations lead to the bonds that cause us to feel invigorated, and they likewise structure the establishment for the perplexing feelings that emerge when we end up missing somebody.

Bonds That Tie Us Together

The associations we structure with companions, family, accomplices, and even colleagues shape our personalities and our perspectives. These bonds are based on the mainstays of:

1. **Shared Encounters:** Minutes spent together make an extraordinary embroidery of recollections that add to the extravagance of our connections. From the commonplace to the exceptional, shared encounters give a feeling of having a place and a shared history.

2 **Sympathy and Understanding**: Connection is supported by our capacity to comprehend and relate to one another. The inclination that somebody genuinely "gets" us encourages a feeling of profound closeness that rises above actual presence.

3. **Weakness**: Sharing our feelings of trepidation, expectations, and dreams with others requires weakness. This receptiveness extends associations by showing our legitimate selves and inviting others to do likewise.

4. **Backing and Trust**: Reliable help and common trust establish the groundwork for enduring associations. Realizing somebody is there for us during critical crossroads encourages a feeling of safety and profound closeness.

5. **Shared Values**: Normal qualities and convictions add to a feeling of arrangement, making it more straightforward to interface on a more profound level. Shared values create a feeling of direction and solidarity.

Effect of Connections on Feelings

The connections we structure are static associations as well as unique environments that shape our close to home scenes. These connections impact how we experience and cycle feelings, including the complicated sentiments that emerge while we're missing somebody.

1. **Intensifying Feelings**: Connections enhance our feelings. At the point when we miss somebody, the profound bond we share amplifies the profundity of our yearning, creating a special mix of sentiments.

2. **Facilitating Depression**: Associations Provide a cradle against dejection. At the point when somebody is missing, the sensation of missing them can at times make us keenly conscious of the void they abandon.

3. **Profound Synchronization**: Cozy connections frequently lead to close to home synchronization, where our states of mind and sentiments line up with those of those we're associated with. Missing somebody can set off an outpouring of feelings because of their non-attendance.

4. **Effect on Adapting**: The strength of our associations impacts how we adapt to missing somebody. The presence of a strong organization can relieve the profound effect of their non-attendance.

5. **Memory and Affiliation**: Recollections attached to an individual can set off a feeling of missing them. The spots, scents, and sounds related to the individual bring out strong feelings that uplift the feeling of yearning.

The idea of association is a fragile dance between presence and nonappearance, between shared minutes and the reverberations they abandon. As we investigate the complexities of missing somebody, we explore the forms of these associations, recognizing their role in molding the feelings that variety our lives.

Chapter 2.

Triggers of Missing You

The sensation of missing somebody is, in many cases, lighted by a progression of triggers that set off an orchestra of feelings. These triggers, inconspicuous or serious, pull at the strings of our hearts, helping us to remember individuals and encounters that have made a permanent imprint on our lives. Understanding these triggers assists us with disentangling the intricacies of why we miss somebody and how these feelings manifest.

Actual Division

Actual division, even for a brief time, can be an intense trigger for missing someone. At the point when the individual we're associated with is presently not within arm's reach, a range of feelings can surface:

1. **Distance:** The geographic space that isolates us from friends and family highlights the longing for their presence, causing each mile to feel like a gap.
2. **Nonattendance of Faculty:** The shortfall of tactile prompts—a recognizable touch, their voice, their fragrance—can strengthen the yearning for somebody.
3. **Day-to-day practice:** The schedules we impart to the individual we miss can summon their nonappearance surprisingly, causing their presence to feel practically like an essential piece of our routine.

Shared Encounters and Recollections

Shared encounters and esteemed recollections frequently go about as triggers, helping us to remember the minutes we've had and making a glaring difference with the ongoing nonattendance:

1. **Commemorations.** Unique dates, commemorations, and achievements trigger a reflection on the minutes we've gathered together to celebrate, highlighting the nonattendance during these huge times.
2. **Places** where recollections were made—a most loved bistro, a recreation area, a traffic intersection—can become close-to-home milestones that enhance the sensation of missing somebody.
3. **Shared Customs:** The shortfall of an individual during customs or ceremonies that were shared can carry their presence to the front of our psyches, highlighting their importance.

Profound Reliance

Close-to-home reliance can be a trigger for missing somebody, especially when they've been a wellspring of daily reassurance or strength.

1. **Partner and Audience:** On the off chance that the individual we miss was our comrade or somebody we imparted our most profound consideration, their nonappearance can prompt a feeling of a close-to-home void.
2. **Emotionally supportive network:** Individuals who offered profound help during testing times became a fundamental piece of our survival strategy. Their nonappearance can cause difficulties to feel overwhelming.

3. **Feeling of Having a place**: Missing somebody can likewise be set off by a feeling of having a place they gave. At the point when they're nowhere to be found, sensations of segregation or separation can emerge.

Understanding these triggers assists us in exploring the profound scene of missing somebody. It advises us that our feelings are interconnected with our encounters, recollections, and the jobs individuals play in our lives. Each trigger fills in as a sign of the worth of these associations, inviting us to consider the effect they have on our close-to-home prosperity.

Chapter 3.

The Brain Research Behind Missing Someone.

The brain research behind Missing Somebody dives into the perplexing exchange of feelings, recollections, and mental cycles that lead to the impactful sensation of nonappearance. This investigation uncovers the hidden components that make missing someone a profoundly human encounter.

Connection Hypothesis and Missingness

The connection hypothesis, created by clinician John Bowlby, gives insight into why we experience areas of strength when isolated from somebody we're connected to:

1. **Secure Connection**: Those with a protected connection style will generally deal with divisions better, as they trust the dependability of their connections and their close-to-home versatility.

2. **Restless Connection**: People with a restless connection style frequently experience increased sensations of missing someone because of their elevated separation anxiety and distraction from the relationship.

3. **Avoidant Connection**: Individuals with an avoidant connection style might make light of their feelings of missing somebody, as they will generally stifle their sentiments and value autonomy.

The Job of Dopamine and Serotonin

The science of missing somebody includes synapses that assume a huge part in our feelings:

1. **Dopamine**: Dopamine, the "vibe great" synapse, is related to joy and reward. It's delivered when we expect to rejoin somebody we miss, adding to the surge of satisfaction.

2. **Serotonin**: Serotonin, which directs temperament and social ways of behaving, can vacillate when we're isolated from friends and family. Decreased serotonin levels could prompt sensations of bitterness and sadness.

Strategies for dealing with hardship or stress and Response

The brain research behind missing somebody additionally uncovers how people adapt to these feelings:

1. **Glorification**: During nonattendance, we frequently glorify the individuals we miss, zeroing in on their positive characteristics and recollections. This romanticizing can escalate the sensation of missing them.

2. **Rumination**: The psyche, as often as possible, returns to recollections and situations affecting the individual we miss. While this can give solace, unreasonable rumination could enhance feelings of pity.

3. **Advanced Association**: In the computerized age, innovation permits us to remain essentially associated. Texts, calls, and online entertainment give a glimpse into the individual's life, possibly reducing sensations of nonappearance.

4. **Interruption**: Taking part in exercises, side interests, or investing energy with other friends and family can go about as an interruption from the feelings of missing somebody.

5. **Expectant Happiness**: Anticipating a gathering can bring expectant delight, which lessens the sensation of missing somebody.

Understanding the mental components behind missing someone reveals the complexities of human feelings and the meaning of our associations. These bits of knowledge advise us that missing somebody isn't exclusively an issue of actual nonappearance; it's a multi-faceted encounter impacted by our connection styles, mind science, methods for dealing with especially difficult times, and close-to-home reactions.

Chapter 4.

Yearning for What Was

The sensation of missing somebody frequently conveys with it a yearning for what was—a longing to get back to the minutes, encounters, and sentiments that have molded our lives. This feeling of sentimentality is both a wellspring of solace and a powerful indication of the progression of time. Investigating this yearning reveals the intricacy of our feelings and the force of memory.

Wistfulness and Its Impact on Missing You

Sentimentality is a strong feeling that interlaces with the sensation of missing somebody.
1. **Embracing the Past**: Sentimentality welcomes us to return to loved recollections, permitting us to quickly remember minutes and feelings that have molded our associations.
2. **Specific Memory**: Sentimentality frequently features positive parts of the past, driving us to long for the delight, giggling, and straightforwardness of bygone ages.
3. **Solace in Commonality**: Nostalgic minutes give a feeling of solace, helping us to remember when things had a good sense of safety and connections were perpetual.

Managing Changes and Misfortune

Yearning for what was can likewise act as a method for adapting to change and misfortune.
1. **Close to home Mooring**: Recollecting how things were at the point at which somebody was available helps anchor us inwardly, making their nonappearance more reasonable.
2. **Managing Change**: Yearning for What Was can help with exploring advances. It gives it coherence and an association with a past that feels recognizable.
3. **Pain and Mending**: Missing somebody frequently goes with melancholy, and returning to recollections of what was can be a stage in the recuperating system.
4. **Representative Importance**: Items, places, or encounters attached to the individual we miss can become images of our yearning, offering a substantial association with what was.
While yearning for what can summon a blend of feelings—solace, bitterness, happiness, and thoughtfulness—it's a demonstration of the enduring effect of individuals and encounters that have touched our lives. This yearning highlights the profundity of our associations, advising us that our feelings are unpredictably woven into the texture of time, memory, and the common moments that characterize us

Chapter 5.

The Specialty of Presence in Nonappearance

The conundrum of missing somebody lies in the specialty of tracking down their presence inside the space of their non-appearance. This multifaceted exchange between memory, feeling, and association exhibits the flexibility of human hearts and our capacity to keep friends and family close in any event, even when they're genuinely far away.

Remaining Associated in a Computerized Age

In the advanced age, remaining associated has taken on new aspects:

1. **Virtual Presence**: Online entertainment, texts, calls, and video talks overcome any issues between actual partition and profound association, permitting us to share minutes across distances.

2. **Visual Updates:** Sharing photographs and recordings makes visual tokens of shared encounters, assisting us in reproducing the sensation of presence through pictures.

3. **Momentary Satisfaction**: Innovation offers the momentary delight of correspondence, empowering us to feel associated with friends and family in any event, even when they're far away.

Keeping up with Profound Closeness

Safeguarding closeness to home despite actual distance is a work of art in itself.

1. **Open Correspondence**: Legit discussions about missing somebody reinforce close-to-home bonds and give an outlet to shared sentiments.

2. **Steady Motions**: Sending smart messages, care bundles, or shock gifts can cultivate a feeling of closeness and care.

3. **Shared Exercises**: Taking part in shared exercises—watching a similar film or perusing a similar book—encourages a feeling of association.

4. **Tuning in and Sympathy**: Effectively paying attention to one another's encounters and feelings creates a space where both presence and nonattendance are recognized.

The Quintessence of Memory

Memory turns into a material on which we paint the picture of our friends and family.

1. **Memory Triggers**: Regular encounters trigger recollections, summoning the sensation of presence even in nonappearance

2. **Living Heritage**: Esteeming the qualities, illustrations, and effects of the individual we miss keeps their embodiment alive in our souls.

3. Groundbreaking Minutes: Extraordinary minutes imparted to somebody become standards that permit us to reconnect with their presence at whatever point we review them.

The specialty of presence in nonappearance is a demonstration of our versatility and the human ability to rise above the constraints of reality. It gives an impression of the profundity of our feelings and the persistence of our associations. Embracing this workmanship permits us to wind around strings of association across the miles, transforming the void of nonattendance into a material where the brushstrokes of memory and feeling make a representation of getting through adoration and friendship

Chapter 6

Turning Missing into Motivation

The ache of missing someone can be transformed into a powerful source of motivation, propelling us to channel our emotions into positive action. This transformation isn't just about finding a silver lining; it's about harnessing the energy of longing and redirecting it towards personal growth, meaningful pursuits, and building connections.

Utilizing Feelings to Drive Activity

1. **Inventive Articulation**: The force of missing somebody can fuel innovative outlets like composition, workmanship, music, or dance. These articulations provide therapy as well as add to self-awareness and self-revelation.

2. **Useful Objectives**: Defining objectives and pursuing them can give a feeling of inspiration. The energy produced by missing somebody can be diverted into accomplishing individual, proficient, or instructive targets.

3. **Developing Appreciation**: Pondering what we miss about somebody can help us develop an appreciation for the effect they've had on our lives. This appreciation can be directed toward thoughtful gestures or helping other people.

Quest for Self-awareness

1. **Self-Reflection**: The contemplative minutes provoked by missing someone can prompt self-disclosure. This mindfulness can drive self-improvement and the advancement of the capacity to appreciate individuals on a deeper level.

2. **Fortifying Flexibility**: Changing yearning into inspiration assembles strength. It trains us to adjust to change, oversee troublesome feelings, and explore difficulties.

3. **Gaining from Misfortune**: The shortfall of somebody can incite us to ponder the temporariness of life. This acknowledgment can motivate us to live more purposefully and capitalize on each second.

Changing Agony into Strength

1. **Strengthening**: Changing missing someone into inspiration enables us to assume command over our feelings and use them as the main impetus in our lives.

2. **Structured Associations**: The void left by missing somebody can inspire us to produce new associations and fortify existing connections. The yearning for significant associations can drive us to connect with others.

3. **Tradition of Affection**: The inspiration brought into the world by missing somebody can add to their heritage. Taking part in exercises that honor their memory propagates their effect on our lives.

4. **Transforming missing into inspiration;** This requires a cognizant change in context. It includes perceiving the profound energy implanted in the sensation of nonattendance and

directing it towards positive undertakings. This change helps our prosperity as well as the association we love.

Chapter 7

Mending and Pushing Ahead

The experience of missing somebody is certainly not a static encounter; it's a way of mending and changing. While the throb of nonattendance can be extraordinary, it additionally holds the potential for recuperation and development. Figuring out the most common way of recuperating and pushing ahead is fundamental for exploring the mind-boggling feelings that go with missing somebody.

1. **Recognizing Feelings**: Recuperating starts with recognizing the profundity of feelings attached to missing somebody. Denying or smothering these sentiments can upset the recuperating system.

2. **Embracing Sadness**: Misery is a characteristic reaction to misfortune and missing somebody. Permitting ourselves to lament, cry, and feel aggravation is an essential step towards recuperating.

3. **Acknowledgment**: Tolerating that the individual probably won't be truly present any longer can be an excruciating but fundamental stage in mending. This acknowledgment doesn't discredit the feelings; all things considered, it assists us with dealing with the real world.

Changing Agony into Strength

1. **Flexibility**: The method involved with mending develops versatility. We figure out how to explore testing feelings and emerge more grounded despite misfortune.

2. **Self-awareness**: The excursion of missing somebody frequently prompts self-awareness. We foster methods for dealing with especially difficult times, the capacity to appreciate people on a profound level and a more profound comprehension of ourselves.

3. **Gaining from Recollections**: Recollections become educators on this excursion. We gain from previous encounters and connections, using them as stepping stones toward a superior future.

1. **Taking care of oneself**: Zeroing in on taking care of oneself is an urgent part of mending. Participating in exercises that give pleasure, practicing care, and sustaining physical and mental prosperity help in the healing process.

2. **Reconnecting with Interests**: Rediscovering leisure activities and interests can be restorative. Participating in exercises that bring satisfaction changes a person's personality.

3. **Inward Strength**: The mending venture reveals internal strength we probably wouldn't have known existed. It helps us to remember our ability to conquer difficulties and track down bliss despite the aggravation.

Embracing Isolation Emphatically

1. **Alone Time**: Isolation can mend It permits us to handle feelings, consider our encounters, and sustain a more profound association with ourselves.

2. **Freedom:** Embracing isolation assists us with creating autonomy and independence, permitting us to track down satisfaction within ourselves.

3. **Time for Reflection**: Isolation offers a space for thoughtfulness, assisting us with acquiring bits of knowledge about our sentiments, wants, and individual objectives.

The excursion of recuperating and pushing ahead after missing somebody is special to every person. A cycle requires persistence, self-empathy, and a readiness to draw in the full range of feelings. As we walk this way, we discover that recuperating doesn't mean neglecting; it implies coordinating the experience into our lives, tracking down importance in the recollections, and utilizing the feelings to make a stronger, more compassionate, and kind self.

Chapter 8

Rediscovering Oneself

The excursion of missing somebody frequently leads us on an equal excursion of rediscovering ourselves. Amidst yearning and reflection, we have the opportunity to reconnect with our character, interests, and goals. This course of self-disclosure is a strong method for exploring the perplexing feelings of missing somebody and discovering a reestablished feeling of direction and satisfaction.

Tracking down Autonomy and Self-Love

1. **Embracing Solitude**: The shortfall of somebody can make space for isolation, a space where we can investigate our contemplations, wants, and sentiments freely.
2. **Self-Reflection:** Finding an opportunity to consider our feelings, values, and life objectives assists us with acquiring clarity about what our identity is and what we need.
3. **Self-Love**: Rediscovering oneself frequently includes practicing self-esteem and self-empathy. It's tied in with perceiving our value and treating ourselves with generosity.

Embracing New Experiences

1. **Trying New Things**: The shortcomings of someone can motivate us to get out of our usual range of familiarity and attempt new encounters that help us learn and develop.
2. **Exploring Passions**: Reconnecting with failed-to-remember side interests and interests can be a happy method for rediscovering portions of ourselves that could have taken a secondary lounge.
3. **Cultivating Curiosity:** Being open to learning and attempting new things sustains interest, a quality that contributes to self-improvement.

Setting Individual Goals

1. **Defining Goals:** The course of rediscovery frequently includes defining new private objectives that line up with our advancing character and desires.
2. **Focusing on Growth:** Objectives connected with personal development, training, professional success, or self-improvement can be strong inspirations.
3. **Creating Meaning:** Laying out and accomplishing objectives provides us with a feeling of motivation, adding to a more profound feeling of satisfaction and fulfillment.

Embracing Change

1. **Adapting to Change**: Rediscovering oneself requires embracing change. Perceiving change is a steady piece of life, and adjusting likewise.
2. **Flexibility:** Developing adaptability in our reasoning and approach permits us to explore the exciting bends in the road of existence effortlessly.
3. **Embracing Growth:** Change and self-disclosure frequently remain closely connected, prompting self-awareness and change.

The most common way of rediscovering oneself is through an excursion of self-empathy, interest, and self-strengthening. Even amid the sensation of missing somebody, we have the chance to develop our relationship with ourselves. As we explore this excursion, we discover that our personality isn't exclusively characterized by our associations with others; it's additionally molded by our inner scene, interests, and the remarkable quintessence that makes us what our identity is.

Chapter 9

Rejoining and Conclusion

The experience of missing somebody frequently conveys the desire to rejoin and the requirement for a conclusion. Rejoining can be a cheerful encounter while concluding is fundamental for recuperating close to home and pushing ahead. Exploring these perspectives requires thoughtfulness, correspondence, and a readiness to embrace the feelings attached to partition.

Reuniting with loved ones
1. **Delight of a Get-together**: Rejoining somebody after a time of nonattendance can be a snapshot of unadulterated satisfaction, loaded up with embraces, giggling, and shared stories.
2. **Revamping Associations**: Rejoining permits us to reconnect on a more profound level, making new memories and reinforcing the bonds that make connections extraordinary.
3. **Valuing Presence**: The experience of missing somebody frequently extends our appreciation for their presence, making the get-together much more significant.

Tracking down Conclusion in Different Ways
1. **Communication**: Transparent discussions can prompt a conclusion by tending to any unsettled sentiments, false impressions, or waiting feelings.
2. **Considering Recollections**: Carving out the opportunity to consider the recollections shared and the examples learned can give a feeling of conclusion as we honor the effect of the relationship.
3. **Making Ceremonies**: Customs, like composing letters or journaling, can be an emblematic method for bidding farewell or expressing our sentiments before pushing ahead.
4. **Tolerating Change**: The conclusion includes tolerating that conditions have changed and embracing the potential for fresh starts and development.
5. **Respecting Feelings**: Conclusion doesn't mean eradicating feelings; it's tied in with recognizing them, figuring out their job, and coordinating them into our account.

An Excursion of Change
1. **Recuperating and Pushing Ahead**: Rejoining and looking for a conclusion add to the recuperating system. They permit us to recognize our feelings, gain from our encounters, and move toward pushing ahead.
2. **Transformation**: The method involved with rejoining and finding a conclusion can change us. It trains us to explore change, convey it effectively, and embrace the advancing elements of connections.
3. **Proceeded with Association**: Indeed, even after the conclusion, the associations we shared keep on holding importance in our lives. They become pieces of our story, forming what our identity is and who we're becoming.

Rejoining and looking for a conclusion are vital pieces of the experience of missing somebody. They address the crossing points of our feelings, recollections, and yearnings. While rejoining can bring a feeling of fulfillment, concluding permits us to turn the page on a part while conveying the illustrations and recollections forward. Through these cycles, we come to comprehend that our associations are rarely really lost; they change, develop, and keep on adding to the embroidered artwork of our lives.

Chapter 10

Embracing the Intricacy of Feelings

The excursion of missing somebody is an embroidery woven from a horde of mind-boggling feelings that recur, framing a mosaic of encounters that shape our lives. Embracing this intricacy requires recognizing the lavishness of our sentiments, tracking down significance at times of nonattendance, and exploring the close-to-home scene with legitimacy and self-sympathy.

Regarding the Huge number of Feelings

1. **Bliss and Bitterness**: The feelings of missing somebody aren't restricted to misery; they envelop euphoria in shared recollections, chuckling, and the expectation of rejoining.
2. **Contradictions**: Embracing intricacy implies understanding that sentiments can be incongruous. We can encounter yearning close to happiness and misery close to appreciation.
3. **Fluidity**: Feelings are liquid and dynamic. They change after some time, answering our encounters, reflections, and connections.

Exploring the Rollercoaster

1. **Highs and lows**: The excursion of missing somebody is a rollercoaster. Having long stretches of profound yearning as well as long stretches of acknowledgment and peace is OK.
2. **Self-Compassion**: Embracing intricacy includes caring for ourselves during moments of weakness. Feeling a blend of feelings without judgment is OK.
3. **Permitting Space**: Allow yourself to encounter the full scope of feelings without stifling or denying them. Permitting feelings to emerge and pass normally is important for the mending system.

Tracking Importance and Development

1. **Illustrations from Feelings**: Every inclination, even the agonizing ones, can offer examples about ourselves, our associations, and our strengths.
2. **Development through Intricacy**: Exploring complex feelings cultivates the ability to appreciate anyone on a deeper level, compassion, and self-awareness.
3. **Extending Associations**: Embracing the intricacy of connections permits us to interface on a more profound level by sharing our genuine sentiments and encounters.

Feelings as an Embroidery of Life

1. **Life's Lavishness**: Feelings make life rich and complex. Each feeling adds profundity to our encounters, making them significant.
2. **Shared Humanity**: Embracing our feelings helps us remember our common humanity. Others likewise wrestle with complex sentiments, creating a feeling of association.
3. **Individual Account**: The feelings attached to missing somebody add to our account, winding around a story that mirrors our remarkable excursion.

Embracing the intricacy of feelings is a challenge to fully integrate into the mosaic of human experience. It's an update that our feelings are substantial, significant, and an indispensable piece of our development. By exploring the rushes of yearning, euphoria, misery, and everything in between, we honor the profundity of our associations and the meaning of the connections that shape our lives.

Conclusion.

The experience of missing somebody is a profoundly human encounter that incorporates a large number of feelings, recollections, and reflections. It's an excursion of intricacy, development, and change—an excursion that explores the fragile harmony among nonappearance and presence, yearning and acknowledgment.

As we've investigated the different elements of missing somebody, we've dove into the feelings that emerge, the brain science that underlies them, and the manners by which we can station these sentiments towards recuperating, development, and self-disclosure. We've perceived the job of association in our lives, how recollections act as strings that attach us to those we miss, and how the actual demonstration of missing somebody can turn into an impetus for positive change.

All through this investigation, we've found that missing somebody isn't exclusively about the agony of nonappearance; it's about the magnificence of shared minutes, the woven artwork of feelings, and the persevering effect of our associations. It's tied in with changing the throb of yearning into a wellspring of inspiration, tracking down comfort in recollections, and embracing the intricacy of our feelings as a demonstration of our humanity.

As you progress forward with your version of missing somebody, recall that your feelings are legitimate, your associations are significant, and your ability to explore the intricacies of yearning and nonattendance is an impression of your solidarity. Embrace the recollections, honor the feelings, and permit yourself to develop through the experience. Amidst missing somebody, you're composing a section of your story that is extraordinarily yours, a story that is woven with strings of adoration, flexibility, and the consistently present embroidery of human association.